Youthful

Longevity

Examining the Concepts of Youthfulness, Aging, and Healthy Aging

By

Mary R. Grant

Table of Content

Introduction 5

Explain the concept of " Youthful longevity, not old." 5

The significance of the notion of youth and longevity 6

Chapter 1 9

The Science of Aging 9

How does aging happen in the body? 11

Factors that affect aging 14

Types of aging (e.g., chronological vs. biological) 16

Chapter 2 19

The Search for the Fountain of Youth 19

Examples from the history of the quest for youth forever 21

Modern methods for staying young 24

The role of diet, exercise, and lifestyle factors in aging ..26

Chapter 3 29

Anti-Aging Products and Treatments 29

An overview of common anti-aging products, such as creams and supplements 32

Evidence for these products' efficacy 35

Risks and side effects of some treatments, like Botox 37

Chapter 4 40

Psychological Aspects of Aging 40

How age affects mental health and well-being 42

Ways to keep a positive attitude about getting older 44

The significance of preserving social bonds as we age ...45

Chapter 5 48

Social Attitudes About Aging 48

Ageism and how it affects older people 50

Attitudes and perceptions of aging that are favorable 52

Impact of media and advertising on public perceptions of aging 54

Conclusion 57

Discussion of the Pros and Cons of the desire to live a youth life 58

Last considerations and suggestions for sound maturing 60

Introduction

Explain the concept of " Youthful longevity, not old."

Youthful longevity is a concept that refers to the desire or pursuit to stay young and healthy indefinitely. The term describes the desire to remain physically, mentally, and emotionally young, often in the face of aging. Being youthful longevity is an age-old human aspiration and has been the subject of many myths, legends, and scientific studies throughout history.

Many people consider staying youthful longevity to preserve beauty, vitality, and energy, and prolong life. This desire has spurred the development of various anti-aging products and treatments, including creams, supplements, and cosmetic procedures such as Botox. However, the pursuit of children forever has challenges. This can create unrealistic expectations and pressures to maintain a youthful appearance, leading to negative self-image and self-esteem. Additionally, some anti-aging treatments may have negative side effects or associated risks.

It is also important to note that aging is a natural process with benefits and advantages, such as increased wisdom, experience, and appreciation for life. So while it's understandable to want to maintain good health and vitality as you age, it's equally important to embrace the natural aging process and find ways to stay mentally and emotionally healthy throughout life.

The significance of the notion of youth and longevity

The idea of youthfulness has been an important concept for individuals and society as a whole. There are several reasons why the idea of staying young is important:

1. Health: Staying young and healthy can lead to a better quality of life and help prevent or control chronic diseases

that are more common as people age. Individuals can improve their physical, mental, and emotional health by maintaining a healthy lifestyle.

2. Beauty: Youth is often associated with beauty, and many want to maintain their appearance as they age. The desire to stay young for a long time can motivate individuals to maintain a healthy lifestyle and engage in self-care activities.

3. Lifespan: There is a belief that longevity can prolong life. While there is no guarantee that an individual can live forever, pursuing youth can lead to a healthier lifestyle and may increase the chances of living a longer life.

4. Social pressure: Society often values youth, and individuals may feel pressured to maintain a youthful appearance or lifestyle. This pressure can be positive or negative, depending on how individuals approach it.

Overall, the idea of staying young can be important to individuals and society as a whole. While accepting the natural aging process is important, maintaining good health and vitality can lead to a better quality of life and increased longevity.

Chapter 1

The Science of Aging

The science of aging is an area of study focusing on understanding the biological processes contributing to aging and age-related diseases. Although aging is a complex and multifactorial process, research has identified several key factors contributing to aging, including genetic and epigenetic changes, cellular damage, and inflammation.

One of the most famous theories about aging is the telomere theory, which proposes that the shortening of telomeres, the protective caps at the ends of chromosomes, contributes to cellular aging and the development of diseases. Related to age. Other theories of aging include the oxidative stress theory, which proposes that the accumulation of reactive oxygen species (ROS) in cells leads to cell damage and aging, and the mitochondrial theory, which suggests that the decline in mitochondrial function contributes to aging and aging. Related diseases.

Research has also identified several factors influencing the aging process, such as lifestyle factors, environmental exposure, and stress. For example, a healthy diet and regular physical activity have been shown to positively impact health and longevity, while exposure to pollutants and toxins can contribute. Cell damage and inflammation.

Technology and medical research advancements have resulted in the development of interventions that can address specific aspects of aging and age-related diseases. For example, medications and lifestyle interventions can help manage age-related diseases such as hypertension, diabetes, and Alzheimer's disease. In addition, regenerative medicine and stem cell therapy hold the promise of repairing and replacing damaged tissues and organs.

Overall, while there is still much to learn about the science of aging, research has identified key factors that contribute to aging and age-related diseases, as well as interventions that can contribute to aging. Can address specific aspects of aging. This knowledge has the potential to improve the health and quality of life of individuals as they age.

How does aging happen in the body?

Aging is a complex biological process that affects all tissues and organs in the body. It is the result of a combination of genetic, environmental, and lifestyle factors and can lead to a decline in physical, cognitive, and functional abilities over time. Several mechanisms contribute to the aging process, including:

1. Cell aging: Cells in the body have a limited lifespan, and as they divide and replicate, they can cause damage to DNA and other cellular components. Over time, this damage can trigger a process called cellular senescence, in which cells stop dividing and become dysfunctional. This can lead to tissue degeneration and contribute to age-related diseases.

2. Oxidative stress: The body produces free radicals as a byproduct of normal metabolism. Free radicals can damage cellular components such as DNA, proteins, and lipids, leading to cellular dysfunction and tissue damage. This process is called oxidative stress and can contribute to aging and age-related diseases.

3. Inflammation: Chronic inflammation is a hallmark of aging and age-related diseases. An injury or infection will typically cause inflammation, although as we age, our immune systems can become dysregulated, leading to

chronic inflammation. This can contribute to tissue damage and the development of age-related diseases such as Alzheimer's disease, cardiovascular disease, and cancer.

4. Shortened telomeres: Telomeres are caps that protect chromosomal ends from damage. Shorten with age. Telomere shortening can trigger cellular aging and contribute to age-related diseases.

5. Epigenetic changes: Epigenetic changes refer to changes in gene expression that occur without altering the underlying DNA sequence. These changes can be influenced by environmental factors such as diet, exercise, and stress and can contribute to aging and age-related diseases. Overall, aging is a complex and multifactorial process involving changes at the cellular, molecular, and physiological levels. While there's no way to completely stop or reverse the aging process, healthy

lifestyle choices like regular exercise, a balanced diet, and stress management can help slow it down. And reduce the risk of age-related diseases.

Factors that affect aging

Aging is influenced by a combination of genetic, environmental, and lifestyle factors. Here are some of the main factors that can contribute to the aging process:

1. Heredity: Our genes play an important role in determining how we age. Some gene mutations and variations can lead to premature aging, while others can contribute to a longer lifespan.

2. Environmental factors: Environmental factors such as pollution, radiation, and exposure to toxins can damage cellular components and contribute to the aging process.

3. Lifestyle choices: Certain lifestyle choices, such as poor diet, physical inactivity, smoking, and excessive alcohol consumption, can contribute to the aging process and increase the risk of age-related diseases.

4. Chronic stress: Chronic stress can contribute to the aging process by triggering inflammation and damaging cellular components.

5. Hormonal changes: The hormonal changes that occur during menopause or menopause can contribute to the aging process by altering cellular function and increasing the risk of age-related diseases.

6. Chronic diseases: Chronic conditions such as diabetes, cardiovascular disease, and cancer can contribute to aging by damaging cellular components and accelerating the aging process.

7. Economic and social factors: Social and economic factors such as poverty, lack of access to health care, and social isolation can contribute to the aging process by increasing the risk of chronic diseases and promoting accelerated aging.

Overall, the aging process is complex and multifactorial and influenced by many factors. While some of these factors are beyond our control, making healthy lifestyle choices and managing chronic disease can help slow aging and promote healthy aging.

Types of aging (e.g., chronological vs. biological)

The scientific community is familiar with a number of different types of aging, such as biological versus chronological aging. The most common types of aging are as follows:

1.   Alteration in Time: The term "chronological aging" is frequently expressed in years and refers to the passage of time. It is the essential kind of maturing and, in general, influences all living organic entities.

2.   Aging biologically: The changes that take place within the body over time are referred to as biological aging. A wide range of factors, including genetics, lifestyle choices, and environmental factors, can influence this kind of aging.

3.   Aging cellularly: The changes brought on by aging that take place at the cellular level are referred to as "cellular aging." Changes in cellular function, gene expression, and damage to cells are all examples of this.

4.   Aging psychologically: The changes in how we think and feel as we get older are referred to as psychological aging. Changes in emotional regulation as

well as declines in memory, processing speed, and other cognitive abilities, are examples of this.

5.   Aging in Society: Social aging is the process by which our social roles and relationships shift as we get older. Changes in employment status, family roles, and social activities are all examples of this.

6.   Senescence: The cellular aging process is referred to as senescence. Alterations in gene expression and cellular damage that contribute to age-related diseases are examples of this.

Over the course of a person's lifetime, there are a number of different types of aging. Making healthy lifestyle choices and managing chronic diseases can help slow the other types of aging and promote healthy aging, but chronological aging is universal and cannot be stopped.

Chapter 2

The Search for the Fountain of Youth

The idea of looking for the fountain of youth has been around for a long time. It's about looking for a mythical or magical source of youth and immortality forever. The desire to avoid the negative effects of aging, such as illness, frailty, and cognitive decline, and to achieve longevity and vitality has fueled this search.

The Greek myth of the goddess Hebe, who had the power to restore youth and vitality, and the Chinese legend of the Peach Blossom Spring, where people lived in perpetual youth and happiness, are two examples of stories and myths about the fountain of youth. People have used alchemy, magic, and a variety of herbs and elixirs to find the fountain of youth throughout history.

The concept of the fountain of youth continues to motivate people to seek out methods for halting or reversing aging today. The search, on the other hand, has taken a more technological and scientific approach, focusing on comprehending the biological processes that contribute to aging and developing interventions to halt or avert them.

Research has demonstrated that lifestyle factors like diet and exercise can have a significant impact on health and longevity, despite the fact that there is still a lot to learn about aging. In addition, advancements in medical technology and research have resulted in the creation of treatments and therapies that are capable of addressing specific aspects of aging, such as cognitive decline and age-related diseases.

The pursuit of healthy aging and longevity is an important goal that can be beneficial to both individuals and society as a whole, even though the concept of the fountain of youth may never be fully realized. It is essential to approach this objective from a perspective that is both realistic and balanced, taking into account the advantages and disadvantages of current interventions and knowledge.

Examples from the history of the quest for youth forever

Anti-aging treatments and products have grown in popularity in recent years as people try to look younger and slow or stop the signs of aging. Some common treatments and products to combat aging include:

Applying creams: There are a lot of lotions and creams for the skin that say they can make wrinkles and fine lines look smaller. Vitamin C, hyaluronic acid, and retinol are typical components found in these products. Moreover, there are a variety of upgrades marketed as anti-aging products, including collagen and cell-supporting nutrients like vitamin E and coenzyme Q10.

Botox: A popular treatment known as botox involves injecting a neurotoxin into specific muscles to temporarily paralyze them and reduce wrinkles.

Botox and fillers: Hyaluronic acid or other materials can be injected into the dermis to give the skin more volume and smooth out lines and wrinkles.

Chemical peels: Compound strips include applying a synthetic answer for the skin to eliminate the top layer, revealing smoother and more youthful-looking skin.

It is crucial to remember that the safety and efficacy of these treatments and products can vary and that some may come with potential dangers and side effects. Additionally, despite the fact that these treatments may target visible signs of aging, they do not address the underlying causes of aging, such as inflammation and damage to cells.

Moreover, it is crucial to remember that aging is a normal and natural process, and while we can take measures to safeguard our health and well-being, we cannot completely halt it. In the end, the decision to use anti-aging products and treatments should be based on the individual's preferences and objectives. It should be approached with caution and based on research and advice from a medical professional.

Modern methods for staying young

Scientific research and medical practice support a wide variety of modern methods for staying young. The following are some of the most well-liked modern strategies for maintaining youth:

Healthy eating: By reducing inflammation, preventing chronic diseases, and promoting healthy cellular function, a diet high in nutrients, antioxidants, and fiber can aid in healthy aging.

Exercise: among the most efficient ways to encourage healthy aging is to exercise regularly. Maintaining muscle mass, avoiding chronic diseases, and improving cardiovascular health are all benefits of exercise.

Stress Reduction: Meditation, yoga, and deep breathing are some ways to deal with stress that can help reduce inflammation, improve mental health, and encourage healthy aging.

Sleep: For healthy aging, getting enough good sleep is essential. Lack of sleep has been associated with an increased risk of both cognitive decline and chronic disease.

Supplements Against Aging: Antioxidants, vitamins, and minerals are just a few of the ingredients in many supplements that claim to aid in healthy aging. Even though some of these supplements might be good for you, it's important to talk to a doctor before taking any of them.

Treatment options: Hormone replacement therapy, stem cell therapy, and gene therapy are just a few of the many medical treatments that can help slow down aging and promote healthy aging. The development of these treatments is still in its infancy, so they may not yet be widely accessible.

In general, there are numerous strategies for remaining youthful that are supported by medical practice and scientific research. The best ways to age well and stay young are to make healthy lifestyle choices and manage chronic diseases.

The role of diet, exercise, and lifestyle factors in aging

Making healthy choices in the areas of diet, exercise, and lifestyle can assist in promoting healthy aging and preventing age-related diseases. Diet, exercise, and lifestyle factors play a crucial role in aging. Diet, exercise, and lifestyle all play a role in aging in the following ways:

Diet: Inflammation can be reduced, chronic diseases can be avoided, and healthy cellular function can be promoted by eating a nutritious diet high in antioxidants, fiber, and nutrients. Contrarily, a diet high in sugar, processed foods, and unhealthy fats has the potential to accelerate aging, promote chronic diseases, and increase inflammation.

Exercise: Maintaining muscle mass, avoiding chronic diseases, and improving cardiovascular health are all benefits of regular exercise. Inflammation and oxidative stress, two factors that contribute to aging, can also be reduced through exercise.

Stress Reduction: Meditation, yoga, and deep breathing are some ways to deal with stress that can help reduce inflammation, improve mental health, and encourage healthy aging. An increased risk of chronic diseases and accelerated aging has been linked to chronic stress.

Sleep: For healthy aging, getting enough good sleep is essential. Lack of sleep has been associated with an increased risk of both cognitive decline and chronic disease.

Alcohol and Tobacco: Smoking and drinking a lot of alcohol can make oxidative stress and inflammation worse, which can make aging faster. Limiting alcohol intake and quitting smoking can slow down aging and lower the risk of chronic diseases.

Generally, going with sound decisions in diet, exercise, and way of life factors is fundamental for solid maturing. These factors can assist in slowing the aging process and promoting a longer, healthier life by reducing inflammation, preventing chronic diseases, and promoting healthy cellular function.

Chapter 3

Anti-Aging Products and Treatments

In recent years, anti-aging products and treatments have gained popularity among people who want to keep their youthful appearance and reduce or prevent the signs of aging. Some common treatments and products to combat aging include:

Applying creams: There are a lot of lotions and creams for the skin that say they can make wrinkles and fine lines look smaller. Vitamin C, hyaluronic acid, and retinol are typical components found in these products. There are many enhancements showcased as hostile to maturing items, for example, collagen and cell reinforcements like vitamin E and coenzyme Q10.

Botox: A popular treatment known as botox involves injecting a neurotoxin into specific muscles to temporarily paralyze them and reduce wrinkles.

Botox and fillers: Hyaluronic acid or other materials can be injected into the dermis to give the skin more volume and smooth out lines and wrinkles.

Chemical peels: Compound strips include applying a synthetic answer for the skin to eliminate the top layer, uncovering smoother and more youthful-looking skin.

It is important to remain cognizant that many treatments and products can vary in their effectiveness and safety, and some may have risks and adverse effects. Additionally, despite the fact that these treatments may target visible signs of aging, they do not address the underlying causes of aging, such as inflammation and damage to cells.

Moreover, it is crucial to remember that aging is a normal and natural process, and while we can take measures to safeguard our health and well-being, we cannot completely halt it. In the end, the decision to use anti-aging products and treatments should be based on the individual's preferences and objectives. It should be approached with caution and based on research and advice from a medical professional.

An overview of common anti-aging products, such as creams and supplements

There are a lot of products on the market that say they are anti-aging. Some of the most widely used anti-aging products are as follows:

Creams for aging skin: Retinoids, antioxidants, and peptides are common ingredients in these products that are thought to reduce wrinkles, age spots, and fine lines.

Sunscreen: One of the most effective ways to prevent premature aging is to shield your skin from the sun's damaging UV rays. It is advised to use sunscreen with an SPF of 30 or higher.

Supplements against aging: Antioxidants, vitamins, and minerals are just a few of the ingredients in many supplements that claim to aid in healthy aging. Even though some of these supplements might be good for you, it's important to talk to a doctor before taking any of them.

Supplements with collagen: A protein called collagen is necessary for healthy skin, hair, and nails. It is thought that taking collagen supplements can help make the skin more elastic and lessen the appearance of wrinkles and fine lines.

Supplements with hyaluronic acid: Hyaluronic acid is a naturally occurring substance that maintains skin's hydration and plumpness. Supplements containing hyaluronic acid are thought to improve skin moisture and lessen the appearance of fine lines and wrinkles.

Devices against aging: Microcurrent devices, LED light therapy devices, and radiofrequency devices are just a few of the many available options that make the claim that they have anti-aging properties. Skin elasticity, inflammation reduction, and collagen production are the goals of these devices.

It is crucial to remember that, despite the possibility that some of these products have advantages, there is insufficient scientific evidence to back many of their claims. The best way to encourage healthy aging is still to live a healthy lifestyle by exercising regularly, eating a healthy diet, and protecting your skin from the sun.

Evidence for these products' efficacy

The evidence for anti-aging products' efficacy varies depending on the product and the specific claims made. The evidence for some common anti-aging products can be summarized as follows:

Creams for aging skin: Retinoids and antioxidants, two common ingredients in anti-aging creams, have been shown to reduce the appearance of fine lines and wrinkles, according to some research. However, there is conflicting evidence, and the effectiveness of these creams may vary from person to person.

Sunscreen: It is well known that sunscreen is effective at preventing premature aging. Using sunscreen with an SPF of at least 30 on a regular basis can help prevent wrinkles, fine lines, and age spots.

Supplements against aging: Many of the claims made by supplements to slow the aging process are supported by scant scientific evidence. Although some studies have suggested that some antioxidants, like vitamin C and vitamin E, may help prevent aging, more research is needed to determine whether or not these antioxidants work.

Supplements with collagen: There is proof to propose that collagen enhancements might assist with further developing skin versatility and decrease the presence of scarce differences and kinks. However, these findings need to be confirmed by additional research.

Supplements with hyaluronic acid: Supplements containing hyaluronic acid are not widely supported by the scientific community as a means of combating aging.

Devices against aging: There is some evidence to suggest that certain anti-aging devices, such as LED light therapy and microcurrent devices, may assist in enhancing the texture of the skin and diminishing the appearance of wrinkles and fine lines. Notwithstanding, more exploration is expected to affirm their viability.

The evidence for a lot of anti-aging products is mixed, and more research is needed to find out if they work. The best way to encourage healthy aging is still to live a healthy lifestyle by exercising regularly, eating a healthy diet, and protecting your skin from the sun.

Risks and side effects of some treatments, like Botox

Many anti-aging treatments are generally regarded as safe, but there are some treatments that may come with certain risks and side effects. The following are some of the potential dangers and side effects of some treatments for aging:

Botox: For minimizing the appearance of wrinkles and fine lines, botox injections are a common treatment. While by and large protected, Botox infusions can cause aftereffects, for example, swelling, redness, and enlarging at the infusion site. Although uncommon, more serious side effects like muscle weakness and difficulty swallowing may occur.

Botox and fillers: Dermal fillers are used to give face areas that have lost volume as a result of aging more volume. Dermal fillers can cause bruising, redness, and swelling at the injection site, despite their generally low risk. More serious side effects, like an infection or an allergic reaction, may occur in rare instances.

Chemical peels: Chemical peels are used to correct uneven skin tone, age spots, and fine lines. Although chemical peels are generally safe, they can also cause redness, swelling, and peeling of the skin. Scarring and infection, among other more serious side effects, are uncommon but do happen.

Resurfacing by laser: Laser resurfacing is used to correct uneven skin tone, age spots, and fine lines. Laser resurfacing is generally safe, but it can also cause redness, swelling, and peeling of the skin. Scarring and infection, among other more serious side effects, are uncommon but do happen.

Before beginning any anti-aging treatment, it is essential to consult a medical professional about any potential risks and side effects.

Chapter 4

Psychological Aspects of Aging

When considering healthy aging, the psychological aspects of aging are essential considerations. While the physical changes that come with aging are frequently the focus, we can also experience psychological changes as we age. Some important psychological aspects of aging include:

Changes in how one thinks: Cognitive function, including memory and processing speed, can change as we age. However, these changes do not always mean someone has dementia or other cognitive problems.

Positive emotions: Aging can affect one's emotional well-being, as some people report feeling more alone, depressed, or anxious.

Alterations in identity: As we move from one stage of life to the next, aging can cause identity shifts. As a result, values, beliefs, and priorities may need to be rethought.

Resilience: Despite the challenges of getting older, many people can remain resilient and adjust to new situations.

Wisdom: Experiences can teach us wisdom as we get older and help us better understand ourselves and the world around us.

It is vital to perceive that every individual's insight of maturing will be special, and there is nobody size-fits-all way to deal with advancing mental prosperity. However, maintaining social connections, participating in meaningful activities, practicing mindfulness and meditation, and seeking support when needed are some strategies that may be helpful. We can encourage a more positive and fulfilling experience of aging by placing a higher priority on our psychological well-being as we age.

How age affects mental health and well-being

Aging can greatly affect mental health. Age can have some effects on mental health in the following ways: Anxiety and depression are more likely: Depression and anxiety may be more common in older people than younger ones. Changes in social support networks, physical health issues, and life transitions like retirement or the death of a loved one could be the cause of this.

Cognitive impairment: Cognitive declines, such as memory and problem-solving difficulties, may occur as people age. Frustration and a diminished sense of well-being can result from this.

Social separation: Retirement, mobility limitations, and the loss of friends and family members are reasons older adults may experience social isolation. Depression and feelings of loneliness can result from social isolation.

Issues with the body: Chronic pain, for example, may be more common in older adults, affecting their mental health and well-being.

Independence loss: Due to factors such as mobility limitations and the requirement for assistance with activities of daily living, individuals may experience a loss of independence as they age. A decrease in well-being and feelings of frustration are possible outcomes of this.

As we age, our mental health and well-being must be prioritized. Examples of this are keeping meaningful activities, staying physically active, getting help for mental health issues when they arise and maintaining social connections.

Ways to keep a positive attitude about getting older

Keeping a positive attitude about getting older is important for your overall well-being. Some ways to encourage a positive attitude about aging are as follows:

Maintain social connections: Maintaining social connections can help alleviate loneliness and isolation and is crucial to one's overall well-being.

Perform physical activities: Physical and mental health can benefit from regular exercises, such as lowering stress levels and boosting mood.

Make mindfulness a habit: Meditation and yoga are examples of mindfulness practices that can reduce stress and improve well-being.

Develop a feeling of direction: Participating in meaningful and purposeful activities can boost a sense of fulfillment and well-being.

Accept fresh perspectives: It is possible to combat stagnation or boredom by attempting new activities, such as traveling or engaging in hobbies.

Show yourself compassion: Self-compassion can help foster a positive outlook on aging by treating oneself with kindness and understanding.

By implementing these strategies, people can maintain their overall well-being and promote a positive outlook on aging.

The significance of preserving social bonds as we age

While maintaining social connections is important for people of all ages, it becomes even more so as we age. As we get older, it's important to stay socially connected for the following reasons:

Reduced risk of depression and isolation: Retirement, mobility limitations, and the death of friends and family members are all reasons older people may experience social isolation. Depression and feelings of loneliness can result from social isolation. Maintaining a social life can help alleviate these emotions and improve well-being.

Enhanced mental capacity: Associating with others can assist with working on mental capability, including memory and critical thinking abilities.

Improved physical well-being: Several physical health issues, including hypertension, cardiovascular disease, and an increased risk of falling, have been linked to social isolation. Physical health and well-being can be helped to improve by maintaining social connections.

Heightened sense of direction: Participating in friendly exercises can give people a feeling of motivation and can advance a feeling of satisfaction.

Opportunities for development and learning: As people interact with people with different experiences and points of view, social connections can offer opportunities for learning and development.

Maintaining social connections is important for maintaining an upbeat outlook about aging and advancing overall wealth. It can give people a sense of purpose, boost their mental and physical health, and combat feelings of isolation and depression.

Chapter 5

Social Attitudes About Aging

Social attitudes about aging can greatly affect how older people feel. Common attitudes toward aging are as follows:

Ageism: Negative stereotypes and age-based discrimination are examples of Ageism. Ageism can significantly impact the well-being of older adults and result in discrimination in employment, healthcare, and housing.

Stereotypes: More seasoned grown-ups are often depicted as delicate, ward, and uncouth in the media and mainstream society. These stereotypes and negative attitudes toward aging can impact older people's self-esteem.

Culture geared toward youth: Western culture emphasizes youth, beauty, and physical prowess, and it is typically youth-oriented. Older adults may experience feelings of marginalization and invisibility as a result.

Neglect of aging: To maintain a youthful appearance and deny the reality of aging, some people may deny or avoid the process of aging. This can hinder people's acceptance of the aging process and the opportunities it presents and contribute to negative attitudes toward aging.

Attitudes of optimism: Positive attitudes toward aging, which emphasize the wisdom, experience, and contributions of older adults, are gaining momentum despite these obstacles.

Aging-friendly attitudes can aid in the fight against Ageism and improve the health of older people. Acknowledging the opportunities and challenges of aging, challenging negative stereotypes, and valuing the contributions of older adults are all examples of this.

Ageism and how it affects older people

Ageism is a type of age-based discrimination that can greatly affect older people. Ageism can affect seniors in the following ways:

Discrimination at work: Ageism can result in workplace discrimination, such as being turned down for promotions or employment opportunities. This can make it harder for older people to maintain their standard of living and contribute to financial insecurity.

Disparities in healthcare: Ageism can also have an effect on healthcare, making treatment and access to care equally. Older people may be undertreated for certain conditions or seen as less deserving of medical intervention.

Social separation: Ageism is the perception that older people are less valuable or interesting than younger people, leading to social isolation and loneliness. This can have a negative effect on mental health and well-being as a whole.

Stereotyping: Ageism can lead to negative stereotypes about older people, like the idea that they're all mentally or physically weak. Older people's low self-esteem and inability to participate fully in society can be impacted by these stereotypes.

Ageism internalized: Internalizing Ageism and developing negative self-perceptions can have a negative impact on older adults' self-esteem and well-being as a whole.

In general, Ageism has the potential to have a significant impact on the lives of older people, resulting in discrimination in employment and healthcare, social isolation, and the perpetuation of negative stereotypes. Alternate adults' well-being can be improved by challenging Ageism and encouraging positive attitudes toward aging.

Attitudes and perceptions of aging that are favorable

Attitudes and perceptions of aging that are favorable can have a significant effect on the well-being and quality of life of older adults. Positive attitudes and perceptions of aging include the following:

Accepting the process of aging: Accepting the changes that come with aging and accepting the process of aging can help people keep a positive outlook on life and feel more empowered to take on new challenges.

Life experiences are valuable: Age-related knowledge and experience can be extremely beneficial to others. It is possible to combat negative stereotypes and foster positive attitudes toward aging by valuing these experiences and contributions.

Engaging in and staying active: Older adults can maintain their independence and improve their overall health by engaging in physical and mental activity.

Building solid social associations: It is possible to combat social isolation and foster a sense of belonging and purpose by establishing and maintaining social connections.

Concentrating on assets: Older adults can maintain a positive outlook on life and continue to pursue their passions and interests by concentrating on their strengths and capabilities rather than their limitations.

Overall, Ageism can be combated, and older adults' well-being can be improved by encouraging positive attitudes and perceptions of aging. Building strong social connections, valuing life experiences, remaining active and engaged, and focusing on one's strengths and abilities are all examples of this.

Impact of media and advertising on public perceptions of aging

The impact of media and advertising on public perceptions of aging is significant. Media and advertising can influence attitudes about aging in the following ways:

Promoting false stereotypes: The media and publicizing can build up bad generalizations of maturing, like accepting that more seasoned grown-ups are all genuinely or intellectually fragile.

Promoting products that fight to age: Publicizing frequent advances hostile to maturing items and medicines can build up the possibility that maturing is bothersome and something to be kept away from.

Making older people appear to be less valuable: The media might portray more seasoned grown-ups as less important or intriguing than more youthful people, adding to Ageism and social detachment.

Underrepresentation of the elderly: Media underrepresentation of older adults can contribute to a lack of visibility and perpetuation of negative stereotypes.

Restricting depictions of aging: The media might depict maturing as a downfall instead of a characteristic piece of the existence cycle; restricting comprehension, we might interpret what maturing can resemble.

By promoting anti-aging products, reinforcing negative stereotypes, and underrepresenting older adults, the media and advertising can have a significant impact on attitudes toward aging. Ageism can be combated, and attitudes toward aging can be improved by challenging these depictions and encouraging representations of aging that are more positive and diverse.

Conclusion

The idea of remaining youthful everlasting has been a subject of interest for a long time, and cutting-edge society keeps esteeming energy and actual appearance. However, numerous factors influence how we age, and aging is a natural process that cannot be slowed down. Although anti-aging treatments and products are popular, their efficacy is frequently questioned, and their use can come with risks and side effects. Generally, Our wellness can be improved by leading a healthy lifestyle, maintaining social connections, and adopting a good view of aging. In addition, it is essential to acknowledge and combat ageism and promote positive attitudes and perceptions of aging in society. We can help combat ageism and promote a more inclusive and positive view of aging by valuing the experiences and contributions of older adults and promoting media representations of aging that are more positive and diverse.

Discussion of the Pros and Cons of the desire to live a youth life

The desire to live a life of youth has advantages and disadvantages, and it is essential to consider these aspects when contemplating aging and the pursuit of youth.

Pros:

1. enhanced physical well-being: Physical fitness, a balanced diet, and a healthy way of life can help you stay healthy and avoid illnesses that come with aging.

2. Improved self-worth: A more upbeat outlook on life can result from having a younger appearance and higher self-esteem.

3. better Chances: Possessing a youthful and vibrant appearance can sometimes open doors to better opportunities in one's professional or personal life.

Cons:

1. Expectations that aren't true: When aging and the changes that come with it occur, the pursuit of youth can lead to unmet expectations and disappointment.

2. Expensive treatments: Treatments for aging are often ineffective and often cost money.

3. Impact on mental health negatively: When aging-related changes occur, the desire to always be young can cause anxiety and depression.

4. exacerbates ageism: Ageism and negative stereotypes of older people can be exacerbated by the emphasis on youth and physical appearance.

Overall, although the desire to live a life of youth has some potential advantages, it is essential to consider the potential drawbacks and accept that aging is inevitable. Instead of aiming for an unattainable ideal, emphasizing a healthy lifestyle, staying connected to others, and accepting aging as a normal part of life may be more beneficial.

Last considerations and suggestions for sound maturing

In conclusion, numerous factors influence our age, and aging is a natural and unavoidable part of life. While it is understandable to want to stay youthful longevity, it is important to recognize the potential drawbacks and concentrate on preserving overall health and well-being as we age. The last thoughts and suggestions for healthy aging are as follows:

Maintain physical activity: Regular exercise can aid in physical health maintenance and age-related disease prevention.

Eat a sound eating regimen: The necessary nutrients for good health can be found in a well-balanced and nutritious diet.

Maintain social connections: Keeping in touch with friends and family can reduce feelings of isolation and loneliness and improve mental and emotional well-being.

Keep a positive attitude about getting older: Accept aging as a natural part of life and concentrate on the benefits of wisdom and experience.

Stay away from destructive things to do: Avoid smoking and drinking too much alcohol, which can be bad for your health and make you age faster.

When needed, seek medical attention: Health issues can be identified and addressed before they become more serious with regular medical care.

We can promote healthy aging and enhance our overall well-being as we get older if we prioritize these things. Recognizing that aging is a journey and that every person's experience will be different is essential. We can live fulfilling and rewarding lives at any age if we accept the aging process and focus on preserving our health and well-being.

* 9 7 9 8 3 8 6 6 8 1 6 9 2 *